Pre-Op Sacred Refresh

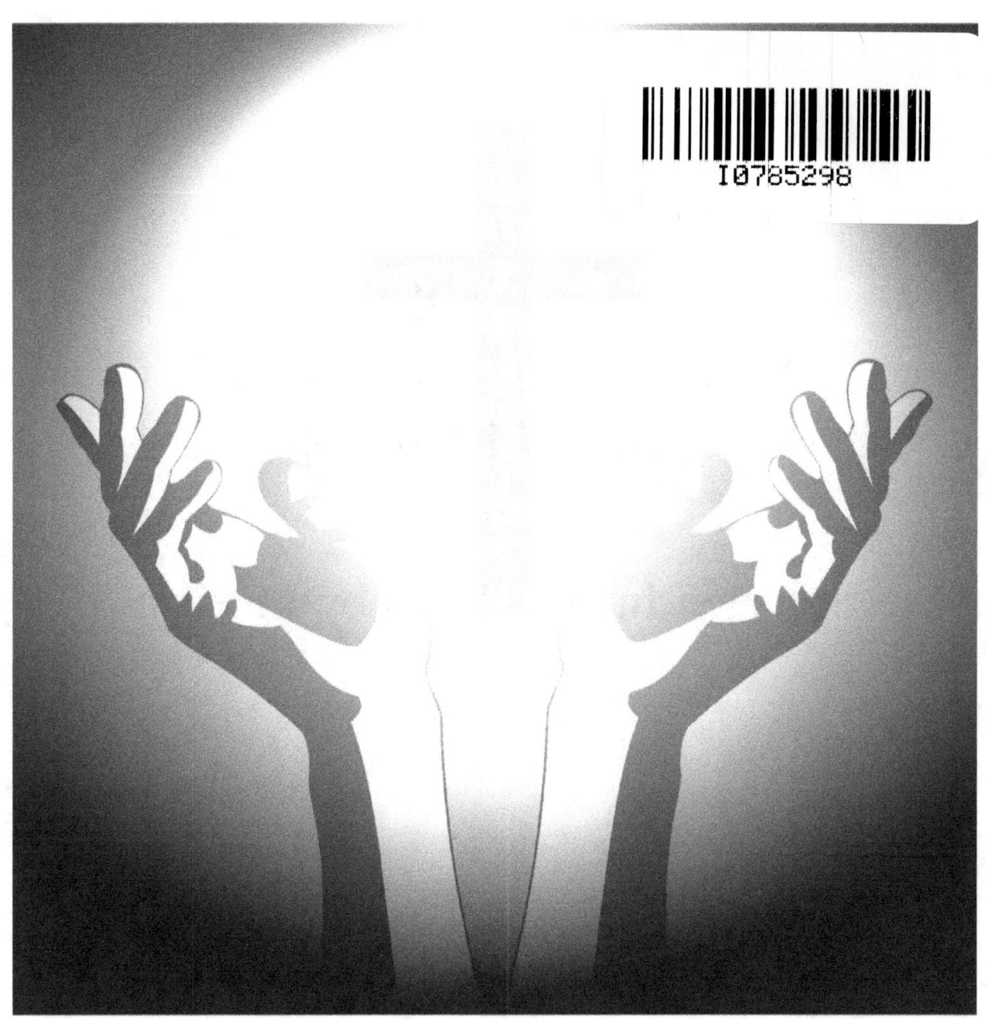

Prepare to Survive!

Rev. Mike Wanner

Copyright
Reverend Mike Wanner
June 21, 2018

Selected Images Used by License

Table of Contents

Dedication

This book is for Surgical Candidates and is dedicated to the Caregivers of all traditions and credentials who will help them. When we think of healing, we usually think of the Doctors and Nurses as their images may be quite memorable from specific experiences in our lives.

These dedicated practitioners of the healing arts are the leaders of the healthcare teams which provide the functionality of medical care. To optimize results, consider including the complete wellness and healthcare community in your thinking as well as your abilities at self-care.

We are of course blessed to be served by dedicated practitioners and technicians of their craft. Unfortunately, many of us do not listen so well and learn enough to optimize our opportunities for ultimate integration of their skills with the human that we each are.

If you listen well, you can learn about the most profound meaning of what your medical practitioners and their teams say and what it means.

Besides all that, more things are under your control than you may have thought. Beyond the physical support of the medical team, we all could benefit from emotional support, mental peace and spiritual uplift that is available from others with skills.

Acknowledgments

I would like to acknowledge the support of the following beings:

Ceil Nuyianes is an Earth Angel who started as a student of mine in Reiki and developed into a friend whose book industry expertise helped guide me in many ways.

Mary E Jay and Teri Goggin-Roberts who have inspired me.

Nancy Russell who was my Integrated Energy Therapy Master Instructor who introduced me to Angel Ariel and the methodology of Heartlinking with the Angels to facilitate the clearing of stuffed emotions and cellular memory.

Stevan Thayer who was my Integrated Energy Therapy Master Instructor Trainer who taught me how to teach others - How to Heal with The Energy of Angels."

My Reiki Masters Rita Hildenbrandt, Hannelore Goodwin, Gary Jirauch, Tom Rigler, Patrick Zigler, Hiroshi Doi, Chiyoko Yamaguchi, Tadao Yamaguchi and especially the founder of Komyo Kai Reiki Reverend Hyakuten Inamoto.

Reverend Ethel Lombardi who taught me the healing power of viewing people as pure light.

Archangels Michael - the Protector, Gabriel - the Communicator, Raphael - the Healer, and the legions of Angels that help the healing process for us all.

This book like others I have written will not be the end all and be all on the subject. I think of my writings as small bridges that can span crevices where a beginning and ending can be seen so eventually many book bridges can be serialized to be an illumed path out of the dark.

The KISS principle (Keep It Simple Sweetheart) is useful in allowing many to find their way through complicated matters. Progress offers a feeling of achievement as one goes along a path from where they were to where they choose to go.

My wish is for you to understand that you are already powerful and can claim access to excellent resources. I invite you to -

ALIGN WITH THE DIVINE

SO YOUR JOURNEY CAN BE FINE.

1 - Illness & Death Anxiety

Once upon a time, I had a friend who carried a fear of the disease that was called Cancer. The panic caused him to be anxious about his health very frequently.

As I understood it, his anxiety carried many visions of Ill health, physical deterioration, and eventual death.

He Focused on what he did not want and manifested it!

The Law of Attraction Can be Used Better!

Please

Focus

Only

On

What

You

Want

2 - Spiritual Preparations Can Help Wellness

Wellness is an optimal way to live so that the best of everything cradles homeostasis which is the natural state of the internal healing system which operates automatically when the body is not under stress. Should stress be an issue for you, free resources can be found at my website http://www.StressReleaseCoach.com

In my earlier books, I spoke about the possibilities for including Reiki and Integrated Energy Therapy®. They can be useful adjuncts to your maintaining your homeostasis.

Should you ever need healing, I invite you to keep notes of all improvements and what is still required as you go through every effort at healing. Please also, Celebrate every little bit of your healing progress.

Progress will likely be slow in the early stages so be sure to capture every bit of development. A celebration of achievement is part of the motivation that you need to keep yourself in the optimal personal position for advancement.

You will be the first one who can claim your progress so do not hesitate to do so. Frustration could quickly set in if you do not recognize the earliest successes and build upon that foundation.

Successes you celebrate will be those that come from your initiative or from any of your caregiving team. Share the achievements with absolutely everybody you see.

3 - Plateauing

You may find that you seem to hit a plateau or a level space in your existence where forward motion is challenging. Accept this as a recommitting spot where you will need to reassess whatever is less than excellent.

Do not study any problems too much for too long. Instead, begin to think and invite creative thought that will pull from joint creative initiatives originating from all who care about you and your progress.

I have been told that the absence of progress in medical treatments can lead to an intense level of frustration which sends one's stress through the roof. I would hope that many could consider any disappointment with their care as a launch pad for the release of a trial balloon into the power of God.

It would be my prayer that the revelations that come through will build sufficient trust for the creation of a bounty of beliefs that can transform your life. Success breeds motivation that can create many more options that can be shared to help many others.

4 - Raising Your Vitality

Forgiveness Is Key

Energy in motion is emotion. Your life force energy is impacted by your feelings.

Taking charge of your feelings can allow you to influence the height or depth of the energy vitality within yourself. When you choose to look at things in an optimal way, you can shift the levels of your internal frequencies higher.

While the ability to do that may sound quite complicated, it is not that hard to do. Just change your thinking, and you move your vibe.

During every day of your life, there are influences around you that can help subtly move your vibration up or down the scale of possibilities. When you feel down because the overwhelming majority of the forces is less than optimistic, your energy and personal vitality can drop to an unhealthy level.

Should you notice that and decide to make a difference in the way that you feel, the actions you take will shift the intensity of those feelings to set a new level. You can pay further attention and monitor the changes and tweak the frequencies until you reach the optimal level you prefer.

Typical emotions that may feel bad are Anger, Fear, Resentment, and Worry. Noticing these things is essential if you want to optimize your options for surgical outcomes

Music can make a substantial difference in feelings by deselecting what is and choosing something else. Another way to make the same move is to shift your perspective from negative to positive.

If you believe the outcome is set and unchangeable, your emotional setting will remain. If you, however, think that change is possible, it becomes so.

Your thinking acts as your life stage setting, and as you reprocess your reasoning, the stage and your life force reset according to the context in your thoughts. I invite you to look objectively at all your challenges and do a 1 to 10 valuation on both sides of everything that causes you any concern. 1 being low and 10 being high helps your perspective to be precise.

Anger is particularly toxic to your options so choosing to release it can be optimal for your wellness, healing, and survival. Will you decide to release it?

Fear can keep you stuck because it may seem that there is nothing you can do. Would you like to release it?

Resentment can be a persistent energy drain and leave you with an empty personal energy battery. Will you choose to release resentment?

Worry is effectively an invitation to an intensity that does not serve you. It helps in nothing.

If you are able to forgive all these threats to your optimal life, You can choose to stand up to your challenges and thrive. The energy that you will find while forgiving will serve your wellness and survival well.

**Invite Yourself
to forgive,
be free,
raise your vibrancy
and optimize your possibilities
for survival.**

5 - The Secret That Makes No Sense

As you go about the investigation of that which is, you can experience many things that seem to make no sense. The illusion of no-sense can be as pure as a perception of elements within a limited expectation of what is.

We can sometimes see things that are not there and not see things that are because we have expectations that may seem helpful at times to shortcut the process. The reality of what we think we know actually has more power over us than the truth that we did not see correctly. Understanding can confirm peace in mind and reality.

This applies to everyday experiences and especially to highly stimulated multi-action scenarios. You have probably heard many witnesses describe an event and their descriptions may sound like entirely different situations.

The mind is influenced by physical, emotional, mental and spiritual stimuli. While we may think that we are aware of everything that we take as truth, we may be in error.

I once worked with a client, and we determined that a significant issue for her was a traumatic episode which happened in-utero. The situation was so extreme because her mother was in a crisis.

The damage was also extreme as it created a dissociative state for the unborn baby which made her prone to splitting again and creating multiple personality states.

By the time I worked with her, there had been two more splits, so it wound up where she had the three alter egos that complicated her ability to understand and cope with her emotional crises.

She also had to deal with her conscious self in the now. I feel that Multiple Personality Disorder can have a dissociative effect similar to Post Traumatic Stress Disorder and that energetic soul retrieval could be the key to the release.

Disassociation is much more common than we might think as most people do it to a lesser degree on a more frequent basis. Nietzsche has been quoted saying "Was mich nicht umbringt, Macht mich starker. (That which does not kill me, makes me stronger.)"

6 - The Gap

There is a crevice between scientific principles and spiritual concepts. It makes little sense for me to try too hard to understand that which I am predisposed to have a difference of approach with but I keep trying as understanding helps me.

Patients, clinicians, and spiritual healers all have different priorities. My priority is that I am writing for those touched with event issues and seek something new to assist them. The approach that I am guided to is spiritual and is in addition to and separate from the professional services that seem to help some but not all.

As the professional services, my suggestions may help some and not all, and that will vary significantly by the engagement factor of the participants. Some will get what I am talking about and others will not, and that is OK. My suggestions are intended for self-empowerment and will not replace the need for professional services at any time.

The scientific analysis by the disciplined professionals does offer wonderfully useful objectivity that can help all clinical efforts and the focus of spiritual modalities. Additionally, active clinical efforts can help to focus on beginning steps, coping skills, and a survival plan.

Hopefully, all suffering from trauma will be invited by caregivers at all levels to be connected to all their support options. Professionals are guided in their work by criteria established within their professional associations.

We live in a litigious society, so professionals are not free to do what they think is best without considering repercussions. They must be concerned about what could happen if they lacked documentation for the care they offered.

While there is sophistication in professional associations' awareness and care plans, all need to remember that each person is unique and that treatment cannot just be an automated process. Government and insurance company efforts are ongoing and necessary to contain cost and ensure the availability of services, but a balance is needed so care is economical while remaining individual.

The unfortunate tendency of control has to focus on that which is tangible and definable which creates an issue in treating individuals with different variables. Patients are each unique, so it is almost impossible to equate one to another precisely so proper documentation is priceless.

7 - Filling the Gaps

There can be many ways to fill the gap. The human experience is diverse and there can be many kinds of sharing that can bring the loving awareness of others to your holistic embrace of all that is available to you.

Objectivity

While practitioners of the healing arts are knowledgeable and disciplined professionals, it is essential for their success to maintain enough distance so they can be objective monitors of the progress of healing or the development of disease so that treatments tweaks can be made as soon as they are needed.

Physical Care

Physical Care is the domain of the Medical Doctor. The general practitioner that we all see is for most of us the gatekeeper for our care. Many routinely surrender responsibility for their treatment to the chosen practitioner.

While professionals take that trust seriously, over time, there has been a cultural dynamic where we surrender too much responsibility to the doctors and don't keep any responsibility ourselves.

Though many of us were taught to believe that doctors are experts, no one is more capable of understanding what we need better than ourselves. Surrendering participation, or putting the responsibility for healing outside of ourselves can actually be detrimental while being full partners with the healthcare team can be empowering and healing.

Consider as if Doctors only have about 25% of the authority that we do. They have a license to practice medicine, and that pertains to just about a quarter of the total care we need. The doctors have the physical area to practice medicine, but we are physical and emotional and mental and spiritual beings.

Unfairly, we have frequently expected doctors to fix everything. They do not have the authority to practice outside their level of licensure. They can help holistically in a medical crisis until the crisis is ended and then our responsibility reapplies.

Most emotional and mental and spiritual elements of us remain our responsibility to integrate into all but urgent circumstances. Unfortunately, many of us do not understand that, and go and sue a Doctor for their malpractice of not taking reasonable care of themselves in a way that is in their long-term best interest.

Emotional Care

The term emotional care means different things to different people, and there are many supporters who are really enablers which support the characteristics of the one being supported in a way that is not healthy.

Just being around and listening to someone is not always helpful to healing and growth. If one encounters a drug addict who needs a fix and wants to help, giving them money for drugs is not the answer. Conversely, this type of support is detrimental.

Emotional support and care are about balance and perspective. It is about weighing all the issues and making balanced, thoughtful decisions that are congruent with one's personal values.

Friends can be most helpful here by planting seeds in the Garden of your mind as to Coach a bit to help identify your next steps on the journey back to health and wellness.

Mind Care

The mind is a complicated and straightforward asset that can bring us understanding and balance. The mind can also delude us into thinking that things are different than they really are and cause us to respond according to what we believe there is instead of what there is in reality.

Positivity is essential to keep one focused and upbeat so that the typical issues of life are dealt with in a balanced way. It is typically not advantageous to overthink the situation that you find yourself within.

You perhaps could find some solace in googling the opposite of your concern. If you can't sleep in the days before surgery, perhaps google How Do I _______________________?

Google is great for a variety of ideas, so please be careful with your wording and selections.

Spiritual Care

The disconnect for many people between the physical realm and the spiritual world can be vast. Many do not realize that the absence of a spiritual connection means that the total support system is not optimized.

God can seem elusive to many people but in reality, God is the constant and we are the ones that may drift away from the blessings that are available to all at all times. When we take the initiative and invite God, the reconnection is immediate and complete.

There is nothing that you have done that is so terrible that you cannot reconnect with your source. The welcome mat is always out. I invite you to plug back into God.

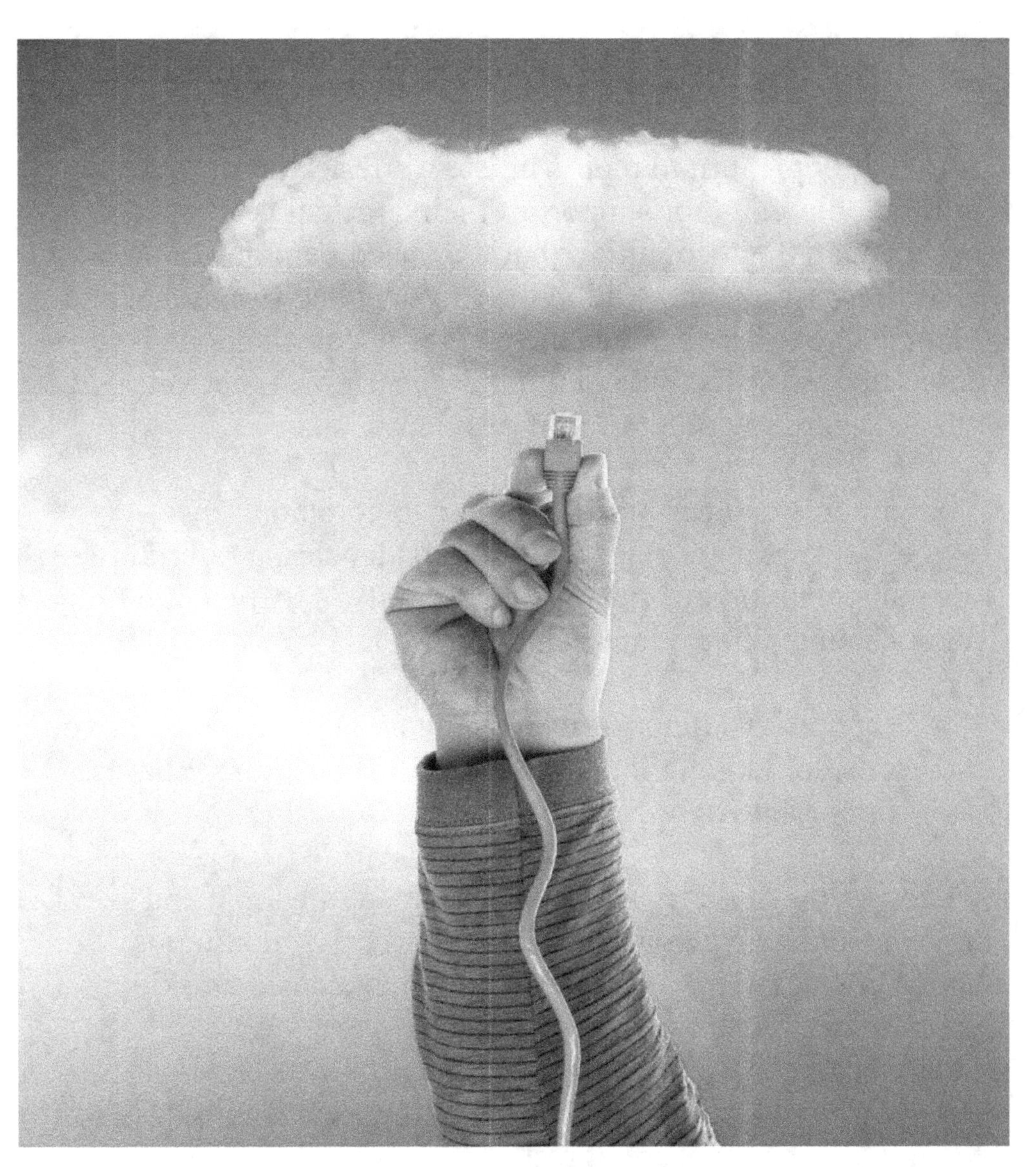

8 - Spiritual Assessment to Refresh

A lot of people turn to their Minister, Priest, Rabbi, Deacons, Spiritual directors for support of their spiritual issues and that has value in the recognition that they need help in that area of their life, just like they did in the Physical and Emotional and Mental levels. The habit of having a safe consultant or counselor has value in beginning the journey of unraveling that which is hard to do for a lot of people.

Your guide's choices may be limited to common sense suggestions, real awareness of your tendencies, a referral to a specialist within your spiritual community, a therapeutic prayer regimen, and clinical intervention.

If a clear spiritual help pathway is not apparent to you yet, you may consider looking into answering the question "What Is Most Important Right Now?"

Perhaps, you could try some writing about the topic and see if there is not some guidance coming forward. If nothing is happening at the tip of your pen, you may consider asking yourself questions about your next step.

Record your questions so your higher conscious mind can visit them later when you are at rest.

9 - Preparing for Surgery & Life After

I do not intend to give you a textbook answer as to how you are to prepare. Instead, this is an invitation for you to settle into the peaceful healing mode that exists when you choose to trust and relax your body, mind, and spirit.

Letting go of the unfairness of it all is enormous. My summary line is "We are where we are." The travel analogy is when you make a wrong turn and wind up in an unknown place. You can sit and wallow in the unfairness, or you can ask directions.

Wherever you are as you read this, I would invite you to find a new way to approach life's challenges. Fear is emotionally devastating. It also affects us physically, mentally and spiritually. I recommend releasing it. You might say that "I can't." Well, you may think that it is true, but I think that you are really saying "I choose Not To release fear."

I invite you now to take your focus off fear, have a little trust and try some things that are new. Follow along with me below:
1. Use all the family, friends and other support systems that you have to determine that what you are doing is the right thing for you.
2. Do all the diligence that you feel is appropriate regarding the time, place, doctors, etc.
3. Do all the diligence that your surgeon has suggested. If you have a disagreement with the doctor, negotiate

a solution. Please don't "yes" the doctor and do what you want.
4. Relax.
5. If #4 is difficult, then get active in taking charge of your subconscious systems by directing your conscious time in the most advantageous way.
   a. Pause and reflect on the many blessings that Have been given to you. Are you grateful?
      1. If you are, offer a prayer of gratitude in accordance with your religious beliefs or if you need help, here is one of my favorites:
         "Thank you, God, for everything
          that you have given me,
         And everything that you have taken away,
         And especially for all that I have left."
         (anon.)
      2. If you are not grateful, please know that you have the power to change your mind and your life at any time.

   b. Think about your surgical team and about how you would like each person on that team to have a really great successful day. If you are comfortable with prayer, you can offer a prayer for them and their families.

   c. Visualize, picture or think pleasant thoughts about the outcome that you would like to see after the surgery. See the desired result clearly and offer thanks for the success.

THE INVITATION IS TO WORRY NOT BUT MAXIMIZE PRAYER, PEACE, LOVE, FAMILY, UNDERSTANDING, ACCEPTANCE AND THE KNOWING THAT THESE MAKE LIFE WORTH IT!

Reverend Mike Wanner
Stress Release Coach
Prayer Therapist
(215) 342-1270
7340 Rising Sun Avenue
Philadelphia, PA 19111
e-mail: mikewann@voicenet.com

Be

At

Peace!

10 - Last Minute Surgery Checklist

___1. Relax your body & mind to ease the stress

___2. Trust in God Almighty Who loves you so

___3. Pray for your Surgical Team & their skills

Poem

When you are ill!

One thing to do still.

Take the time right away,

Pray for your Doctor's Health to stay.

Doctors need time to work on you,

Your prayers work on doctors too.

{From - Reiki Journaling From Japan}

The Greatest Physician is God the Almighty!

If you want help, just ask!

{From - Reiki Journaling From Japan}

11 - Wrap Up

As You Prepare to Optimize Your Readiness
For Medical Care.

Don't Go Alone!

Take the Hand of Your Creator
And Feel Connected!

Offer Thanks for Blessings Already Lived

Expect to Be Blessed
By God's Will

We May Walk Separate Paths
At Separate Times
All Paths Can be Divine
When We Unify with God
In The Here or the Hereafter.

May You Walk Stress-Free and Blessedly

{Note}
The Last Chapter is a Poem of a Friend's Journey.
You can substitute Healing, Prayer or other words that align
with your Spiritual Practice in place of the word Reiki.

12 - My Friend is Fine
{Poem}

My friend was sick once upon a time.
Now she is really doing fine.

She was so smart.
Her healing, she did start.

The Doctors were so great.
Counseling, prescribing, agreeing to a little wait.

She knew what she could do.
She knew what she couldn't too.

A healing team she started,
Her illness shortly parted.

With what all did she deal?
With all, that helped her heal.

She did the Reiki every day.
She gave her body the right pay.

Every week, she had a session.
Doctors, healers in succession.

Her family history.
Offered some mystery.

Was the family strain,
contributing to her pain?

The question put her to the test.
The answer was really the best.

It told her clean and true.
Here, she had to deal too

.

What was painful to do.
Was an answer true.

Her relationship with God came up to.
For a long time, she didn't know what to do

There was a gap,
as if they had a spat.

Since it wasn't that,
she put love in the gap.

Free of all these things,
her energy level sings.

This friend of mine is really doing fine.

Rev. Mike Wanner, Copyright 11/14/2001 Written in Tokyo
from "Reiki Journaling from Japan." mikewann@voicenet.com
7340 Rising Sun Ave. Phila. PA 19111 215-342-1270

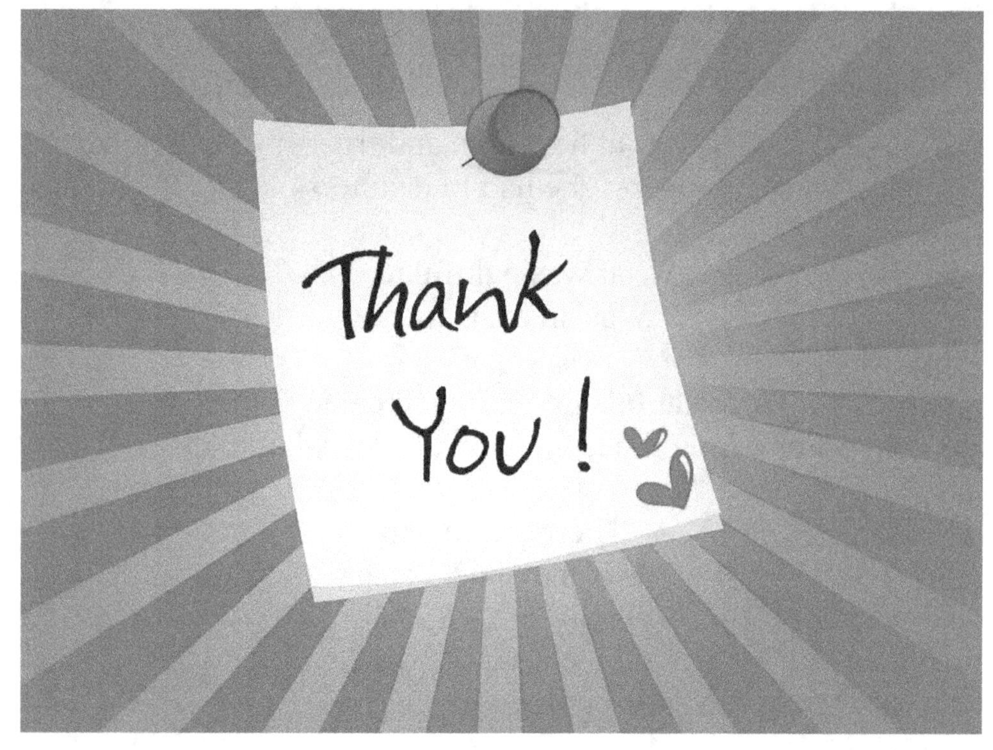

For
Considering
These
Ideas

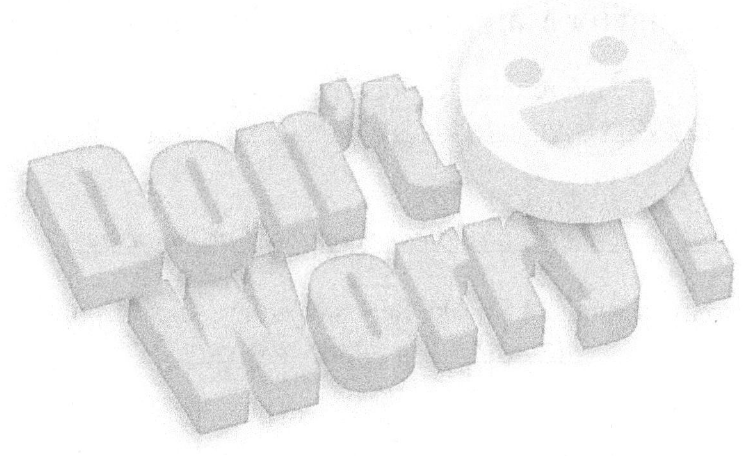

Ever

It Does Not Help Prayer Still Does!

Resource: http://Create-A-Prayer.com

15 - Books Category Resources
at <u>www.Amazon.com</u>

Distant Healing (or Mail List) e-mail mikewann@voicenet.com

Veterans Healing Six Pack plus 2
http://angelraphaelspeaks.com/healing-books/veterans/

PTSD Power Pack
http://angelraphaelspeaks.com/healing-books/ptsd/

Angel Raphael Speaks Series & Other Angel Books
http://angelraphaelspeaks.com/

Reiki
http://angelraphaelspeaks.com/healing-books/reiki/

Children
http://angelraphaelspeaks.com/healing-books/children/

Emergency Medical Kindness
http://angelraphaelspeaks.com/healing-books/emergency-medical-kindness/

Cancer
http://angelraphaelspeaks.com/healing-books/cancer/

Addictions
http://angelraphaelspeaks.com/healing-books/addictions/

Miscellaneous Healing
http://angelraphaelspeaks.com/healing-books/misc-healing/

Prison Books - 50+ Prison Books
http://angelraphaelspeaks.com/prison-books/

16 - Angels Please Prayers

Addict's

Angels of Healing Selected
Help Me to Stay Directed
Come To Me From The Sky
I Am Ready to Succeed Not Try
If I Don't Invite You In
I Might Not Win
I Have Been Lost For Too Long
Help Me To Stay Strong

Alcoholic's

Angels of Healing On High
Help Me to Stay Dry
Come To Me From The Sky
I Am Ready to Succeed Not Try
If I Don't Invite You In
I Might Not Win
I Have Been Lost For Too Long
Help Me To Stay Strong

From

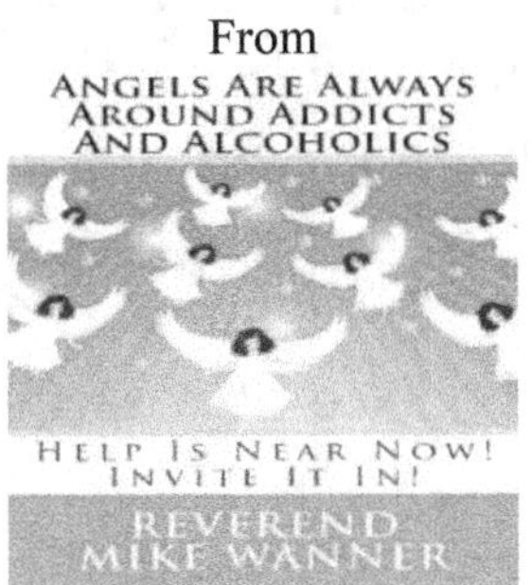

http://AngelRaphaelSpeaks.com/AAAAAAA/
The Link Above Has the Core Messages from the book on drop-down pages.

17 - Private Channeling

Angel Raphael Speaks a series of free messages that are channeled through Reverend Mike Wanner for the Highest good and Highest Healing of all concerned.

Many questions arise about Reverend Mike doing private channeling, and he does help with that so E-mail him.

Reverend Mike is available worldwide as a psychic channel, emotional release facilitator, spiritual energy practitioner & teacher, and public speaker. He looks forward to meeting you soon! Email - mikewann@voicenet.com 215-342-1270

Private Spiritual Readings/channelings or Spiritual Healing Sessions: Telephone or in person.

Rev. Mike is available for individual, intuitive one-on-one sessions with you, his Guide Family, and your Guides. He helps by offering clarity on emotional situations about your life, your purpose, your spirituality, and your release of stuffed emotions and cellular memory.

Connect to the love of your Guides today!

For more information, Please visit

http://angelraphaelspeaks.com/channel/

18 - Reverend Mike Wanner

Rev. Mike Wanner started his spiritual and ministerial studies with Reiki in 1993 and had studied seven styles of Reiki in the U.S., Japan, Canada, Denmark and Australia. He is certified to teach. He became certified to teach Integrated Energy Therapy in 1999 and co-taught the first IET class of the new Millennium. Mike began dowsing in 2001.

Ordained as an Interfaith Minister of the Circle of Miracles Ministry and a Metaphysical Minister of the International Metaphysical Ministry, Rev. Mike practices and teaches spiritual energy therapies in the Philadelphia Area.

Rev. Mike holds ministerial degrees from the University of Metaphysics and the University of Sedona. He is a Pastoral Care Associate at Jefferson - Frankford Hospital. He taught at the National Academy of Massage Therapy and Health Sciences.

Rev. Mike was a faculty member of the Medical Mission Sister's Center for Human Integration's School of Integrated Body/Mind Therapies in Fox Chase, Philadelphia, PA for twelve years.

For a complete Biography, Please visit
http://ReverendMikeWanner.com/Bio

www.ingramcontent.com/pod-product-compliance
Lightning Source LLC
Chambersburg PA
CBHW070104260726

48658CB00002B/972